A STEP TO ACTIV8TION

VOLUME 1

BEN GREEN

Author: Ben Green Title: A Step To Activation
ISBN: 978-1-99972-235-7 Category: Health /Children / Self-help

Publisher: Breakfree Forever Publishing Division of Michelle Watson
51 Gospatrick Road London N17 7EH www.break-freeforever.com

Dedication

I have been on a 15 year journey dedicating my life to helping others. Some might say I have a gift in what I do, however I just want to make a difference in this world and help as many people as I can in doing so.

At the age of 31, I have been fortunate enough to have helped hundreds of children with different backgrounds by equipping them with new approaches to finding their inner greatness!

I would like to dedicate this book to all the children I have assisted over the years, and to the children who are about to go on this new journey of self-discovery.

Finally, I would like to thank my family and friends who have stuck by me on this journey and believed in my vision.

Acknowledgements

The completion of this book could not have been possible without the participation and assistance of so many people. Their input and feedback to help shape this unique book and drive my vision to the next level are greatly acknowledged.

I would like to give special thanks to:

Miss Rebecca Green & Mrs Sjeane Brzuszkiewicz who have been the driving force with me in the process of developing the book.

Mr Stephen Timms (Illustrator) who has created the fantastic illustrations and brought the book to life.

Michelle Watson (Book Publisher & Founder of Breakfree Forever Publishing), your guidance along this journey has been phenomenal. A massive thank you to Sabrina Ben Salmi, your mentorship over the past two years has been phenomenal

From the bottom of my heart I thank you all.

Ben

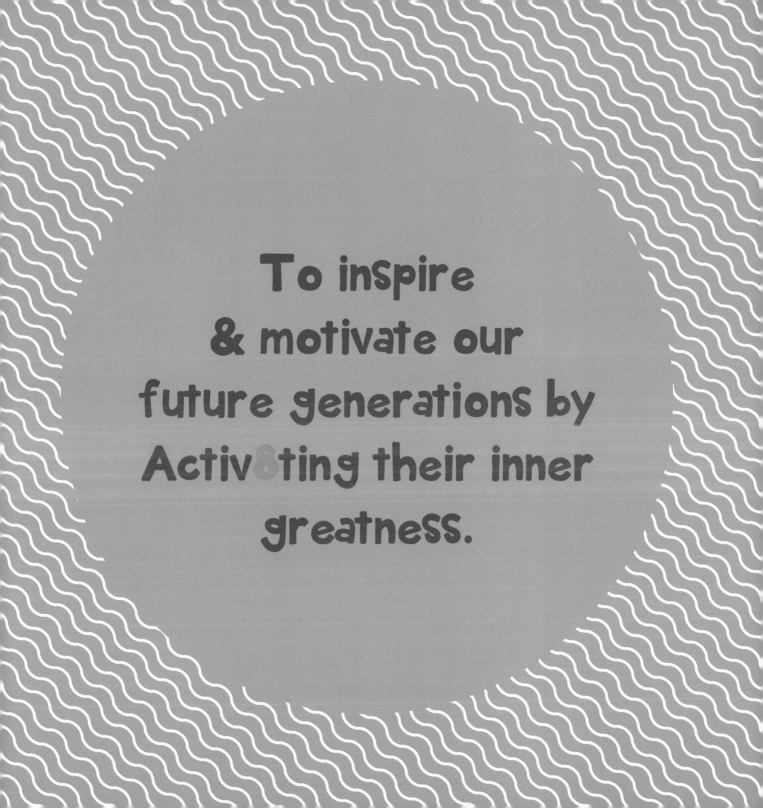

To inspire & motivate our future generations by Activ8ting their inner greatness.

Foreword

As recognition of the importance of
mental health grows amongst all those
involved in the raising of our children, as
well as the broader public - thanks in no small
part to the 'Young Royals' - this book could not have
come at a better time.

Ben's vision for an approach to children's well-being that
encompasses all aspects of a healthy life, from nutrition
to exercise, to understanding and managing feelings, is
compelling. He has created a book that coaches youngsters in
an accessible, inclusive and engaging way, empowering them
to adopt a 'can do' mind set and a 'let's do' approach.

This book will be invaluable for all those looking for a
practical way to support children in developing habits that
become the foundations of a healthy, happy and fulfilling
life.

Melanie Whitfield Head Teacher BA hons, PGCE, NPQH

Melanie has twenty seven years of teaching
experience in both mainstream and SEN schools.
Melanie has been Head Teacher in both settings.
At present Melanie is a Head Techer of a
new school which she has taken pride
in establishing for children with
autism in Cheam.

Contents

Introduction

Well done for getting this far! You are about to go on a fun journey of self-discovery!

Throughout this book, you are going to come across different topics, which will help you understand more about yourself and others. Sometimes we can focus so much on improving everything around us, that we forget to improve ourselves. Just remember, you are very special, and you should never change who you are to fit into another group. We want you to feel confident in your abilities. Keep developing what you are good at and work on areas which need improving.

We want to transform you into an Activ8 Hero! so that you can Inspire others to be Motivated when times get tough and to show your Dedication by sticking to the journey.

Inspir8tion

+

Motiv8tion $=$ Activ8tion

+

Dedic8tion

We are here to help you!

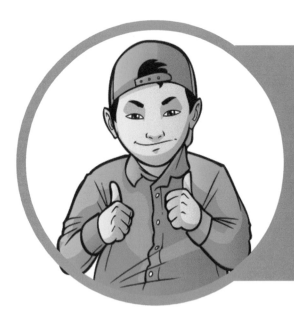

Hi! It's so great to see that you are about to embark on this fun journey with me. I use a wheelchair but I can still do a lot of things without using my legs. In this book I discovered that, the key to forward is being consistent, being honest with yourself and asking for help when you need it. Go and get them champ!

Charlie

Noah

Hello there, nice to meet you!
You are going to get so much out of this book. It really helped me understand the importance of taking care of your body and mind. Before I became an Activ8 Hero, I was very quiet and didn't really talk to many people because I was very shy. Look at me now. I am an Activ8 Hero who is ready to help you on this amazing journey.

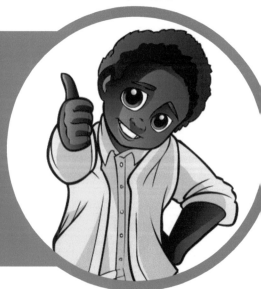

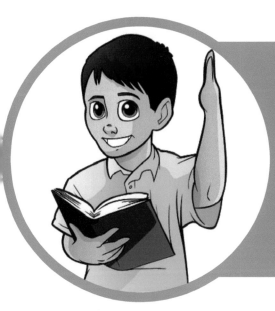

My name is George and I love to learn. I have had so much fun through each chapter of this book: I found out so many cool things. Here is some advice, if you don't understand a certain part of the book the first time you read it, read it again or read it with a grown-up, it will really help you. I also discovered that, doing the activities over and over again helped as well, as practice makes progress.

George

Ana

I'm so excited for you! This book has given me the knowledge to understand my feelings and emotions (feelings and emotions are explained in the book, so don't worry if you don't know what they are). This has helped me understand my friend's emotions and feelings as well. Just remember to take your time going through the activities. It is important to remember that everyone works and learns at their own pace, so take your time, have fun and enjoy the journey.

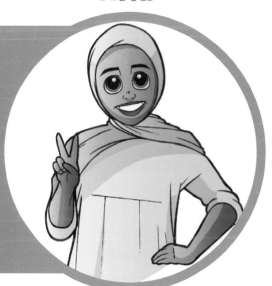

Meet our activ8 Heroes

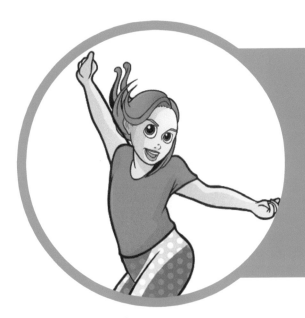

Hi there! I am Amy and I love keeping fit. I also enjoy exercising with friends. There is something really exciting in this book that will help improve your fitness levels. Don't skip through any page; work through the book gradually because they are all important steps to help you become an Activ8 hero.

Amy

Bella

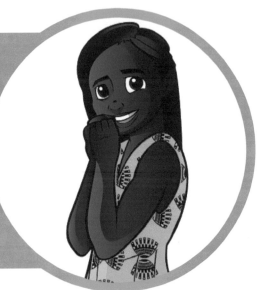

Hi! I'm so excited for you! This book has a lot of great information for you to learn from. Once you have read the first chapter, there is a reflection journal at the back of the book. Just answer the questions honestly and jot down what you feel. Try your best to do this every evening for the next 8 weeks as it will show you how far you have come.

GOOD LUCK!

Let's get ready to take our first step to Activ8tion and have some fun exploring!

Are you ready?

Ready, Steady . . . GO!

Reflection is something we do every day, but sometimes we do not do this in the correct way.

When we reflect, it's often for the purpose of thinking back on something that has already happened. When we reflect on our day, we become aware of the positive and exciting things that happened.

We will also be aware of the negative things that happened, and we will be able to think of better ways of managing a situation when faced with the same circumstance in the future. Reflecting is good as it can help you identify your strengths and areas of improvement. This can help to create new questions and to gain more information to power your brain.

Let me share some different ways you can reflect. The most common way of reflecting is through writing your thoughts down at the end of each day, this can help you improve your emotions. Sometimes, we hold on to our emotions because we feel embarrassed of showing them to other people, family or friends. Sometimes, this creates negative emotions. Reflecting on your day by writing down your emotions on a piece of paper can help you be more aware so you can make a positive change. One of my friends wasn't very good at writing. At the end of each day, he told his mum about his day and she wrote it down for him. Another great way of reflecting on your day is by drawing pictures. I found out that I am very creative whilst doing this and now I have another positive hobby.

Can you think of any other ways of reflecting? Write them in the thought bubbles.

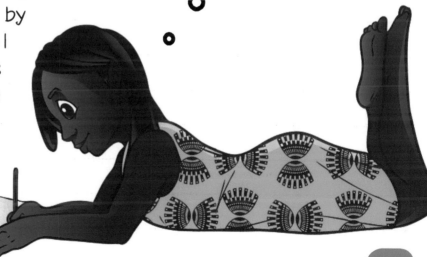

15

There was a time when negative experiences held me back from achieving my goals. One time, I was asked to run around the playground without stopping and I couldn't do it. I was scared to try. I didn't want to feel like that ever again.

Have you ever felt like this?

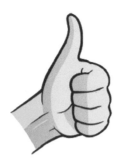
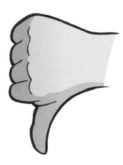

Would you like to share with us a little more about your experience?

_____

_____

_____

_____

_____

_____

_____

What I realise now is that some of the negative experiences we have can be made better by reflecting on them. Once I was able to explain what happened and how it made me feel, I could see what I needed to do to try and improve this experience.

Why don't you give this a try?

Negative experience	How did I make this better?
• Not being able to run a full lap on the playground whilst my classmates were watching.	• I went to the local park with my Dad and practised running around the football pitch. This improved my fitness levels and confidence, and guesses what!? I very easily completed the lap around the playground!

Let me know how your day has been for the next 8 weeks. At the back of the book, you will find an 8-week reflective journal. Your mission is to fill this journal every day.

Top Tips

 When you are writing a reflection, there is no wrong answer. Do not be afraid to express your emotions.

 Try and create a routine for your day. The perfect time to reflect is when you have completed all the tasks you had set out to complete for that day. You may find yourself repeating some journal entries. This is ok. You don't have to feel different every day.

 Remember **YOU ARE GREAT!**

When I was growing up, I loved trying new things and going to new places. This gave me emotions of excitement, joy and sometimes it made me feel nervous as I wasn't quite sure what to expect. I was told nerves are good as it shows you care about what you were about to do. Have you ever felt like this?

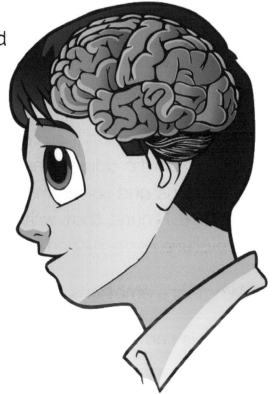

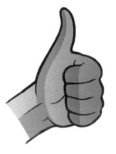 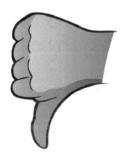

Would you like to give us an example?:

_____

_____

_____

_____

_____

_____

Feelings and Emotions

When I was your age, I was surrounded by a lot of adventures that I loved doing and others that I didn't quite understand. This brought about different feelings and emotions.

Sometimes, I didn't quite understand why I felt a specific way, and it was hard to explain to adults and others how I felt. This made them ask me even more questions and sometimes their questions made me react in a way that they did not like. I found that writing down my experiences on a piece of paper or drawing a picture really helped me to explain how I was feeling.

What are emotions and feelings and what is the difference between the two?

Here is something quick to help you understand.

> **Emotions are what we feel first on the inside and feelings are the words and actions we use to express our emotions.**

The first thing I want you to know is that everyone has feelings and nobody can help having them!

We feel different things everyday depending on the different activities we do.

What are you feeling right now as you read this?

_____
_____
_____
_____
_____
_____
_____

Are you curious and/or hopeful that you'll learn something about yourself?

Are you bored because this is something you have to do, or are you happy because it's something you enjoy?

_____
_____

Feelings and Emotions

Whatever it is, emotions like these are normal and they give us information about what we're experiencing and help us understand how to manage ourselves.

Emotions come and go. Most of us feel many different emotions throughout the day. Some emotions last for just a few seconds while others might last longer. We sometimes feel happy when we see someone we love. We can also feel sad when you lose something important or angry when someone hurts our feelings. Emotions can sometimes also be very strong and other times not so much. Emotions can also be very confusing.

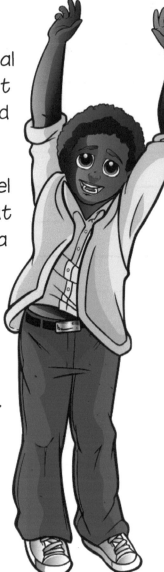

Have you ever experienced some of these feelings?

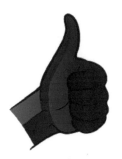 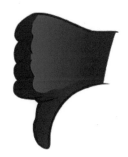

Would you like to share an example of this and what is it that made you feel that way?

_____

_____

_____

_____

_____

Some emotions are positive – for example: feeling happy, loving, confident, inspired, cheerful, interested and grateful.

Other emotions can seem more negative – for example: feeling angry, resentful, afraid, ashamed, guilty, sad and worried.

Both positive and negative emotions are normal.

Feelings and Emotions

Did you know that you have different chemicals in your brain that make you feel different emotions? How cool is this! When you are feeling a strong emotion, it means a certain type of chemical is working in your brain!

Here is your first task.

Below is a list of words.

Can you categorise them in the table according to whether they are positive or negative feelings?

Happy, Sad, Confused, Bored, Angry, Excited, Relaxed, Surprised, Frustrated

Positive	Negative

Now, look at the Activ8 Heroes' faces below and tell us what emotion you think match their facial expression:

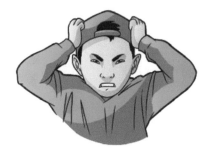

....

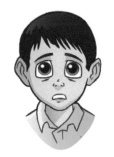

....

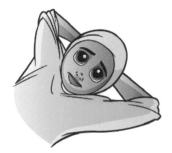

....

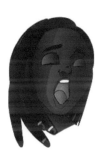

....

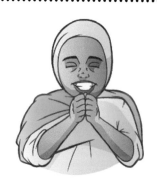

....

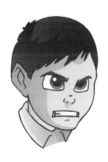

....

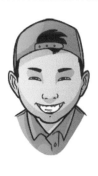

....

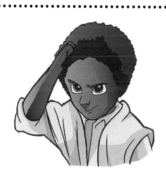

....

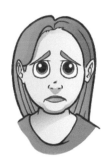

....

Top Tips

 If you are experiencing any negative emotions, try and talk to an adult about why you feel this way. If this is difficult, write it down or draw a picture to express how you feel.

 Sometimes, when we experience a negative emotion, we can act in a way that can upset the people around us. Work with an adult to channel these negative emotions into something positive.

Getting up in the mornings can sometimes be difficult.

This can be for many different reasons. However, it is very important to begin your day in a positive way as this will put you in a great mind set.

To get you up and motivated in the morning, I want you to try my 8 steps to Activ8tion. Let's start the morning off with positivity and fun:

Follow steps 5,6,7 in any order. This varies because different people have different lifestyles.

1. As soon as you wake up, get straight out of bed – if you lay there for too long, you risk falling back into sleep, which will possibly make you feel stressed and anxious when you wake up again.

2. Look at yourself in the mirror and repeat these three sentences:

   I am **GREAT**
     I am **STRONG**
       I am **HAPPY**
      SAY IT LIKE YOU MEAN IT!

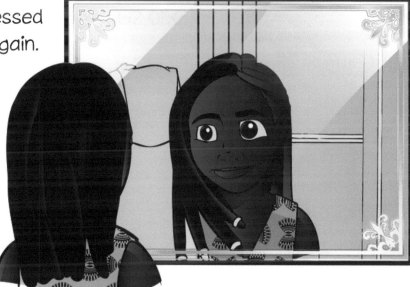

3. Loosen up and shake those muscles

4. Wake your body up with these three simple exercises:

X 10 Star Jumps   **X10** Punches   **X10** High Knees

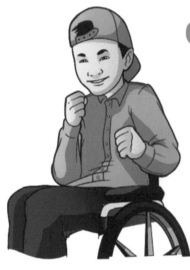

Charlie My alternatives -

X10 punches

X10 overhead punches

X10 Side arm raisers

(Repeat 3 times)

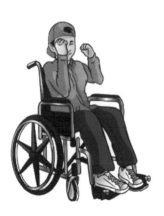 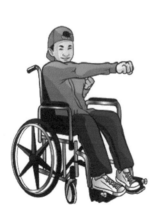 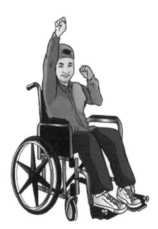 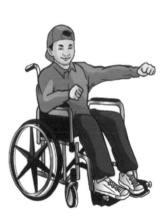

Emotion comes from motion

5. Breakfast is such an important meal; make sure you provide your body with energy to start off your day well.

6. Spread the love. Tell each person who is special to you that you love them or give them a compliment.

7. Shower and get dressed. Most of us enjoy doing something extra to get us going in the morning. What do you enjoy doing? _____

8. What can your last step be? Sit down and have a discussion with an older family member. Remember this is your last step to Activ8 your day, make it special.

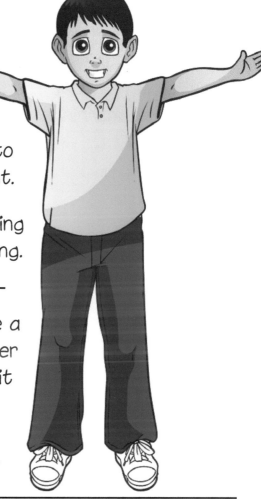

_____

_____

_____

_____

_____

Top Tips

 Make sure you have fun while doing the steps; you can even get the adults to participate. I understand that it will be difficult to do all 8 steps during some mornings. However, try and follow a consistent routine to see the benefits.

Well-being covers every aspect of your life. It's the feeling of being comfortable, healthy and happy with what surrounds you.

There are a lot of elements in my life that make me happy. They make me want to share my experiences, thoughts and give back to others.

Here is a task for you to complete. You can do this by yourself or with a grown up.

Can you list 5 things that make you happy in your life?

1. _____

2. _____

3. _____

4. _____

5. _____

Here are some examples of what make us happy in our lives:

Family

School

Pets

Give yourself a big well done for completing this task!

What is well-being?

How do you feel?

Write down your feelings/or draw a picture to tell us:

Writing things down helps us to understand ourselves better by seeing something rather than thinking about it. It helps us to recognise our feelings more clearly. For example, what makes us happy or sad or frustrated.

Let us explore this a little bit more

From your list of things that make you happy, select 3 and write down what exactly makes you happy about them. For example:

My family makes me happy because we communicate well, we eat dinner together and go on family outings together.

1. _____

_____

_____

2. _____

_____

_____

3. _____

_____

_____

Wow! You have written down some great answers.

Thank you for sharing this with us.

When we look further into our thought process, we can discover amazing things about ourselves sometimes. Just remember, everyone is different in their own special way. Don't be afraid to express this.

Could you tell us how you feel after completing this activity (draw a picture)?

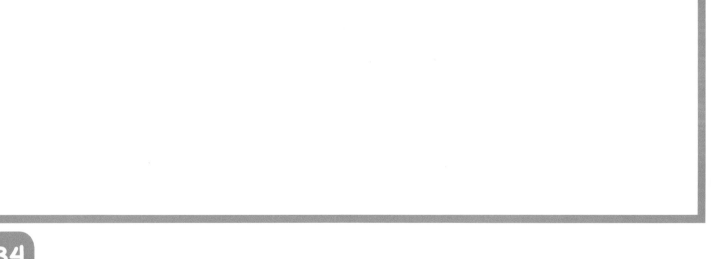

Top tips

 Attempt to do new and positive activities that help you to feel even better than you already are.

 Build and maintain good relationships with other people.

 If you are happy, don't be afraid to show it!

What can affect our well-being?

In life, we sometimes come across things that make us upset, sad, confused and angry. This can have such a big impact on our progress in the right direction. Have you ever felt like you don't fit into a certain group, you stand out in a crowd, or you feel embarrassed to say how you feel out loud?

You are not alone in this, I know that these feelings are not nice and sometimes, we cannot work out why we feel this way.

What can have a negative impact on your well-being? Here are some examples:

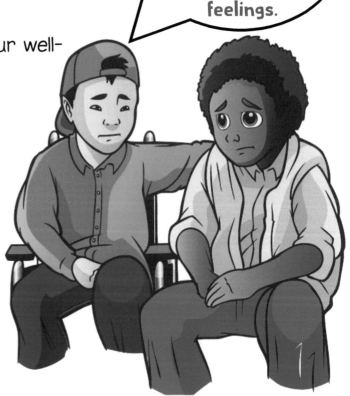

It is okay to talk about how you are feeling because, everyone has feelings.

Bullying

Arguing with friends

Peer pressure

Lack of exercise

Not meeting Expectations

Eating too many treats

Not enough sleep

Name calling

Can you add any more to this list? This can be something you have experienced or something you are aware of, or maybe seen someone else say or do.

What else can affect someone's well-being?	Can you explain?

How do you think you can improve the things that affect your wellbeing?

_____

_____

_____

_____

_____

What can affect our well-being?

Is there anything affecting your well-being?	How is it making you feel?	How do you think you could change this?

What does it mean to you when we say you are in charge of your well-being?

What would you like to change to improve your well-being?

Top Tips

 If you come across anything that brings up negative emotions, try and speak to an adult about it as this can affect your wellbeing. There are a lot of people you can talk to who will provide support; for example, parents, carers and a school teacher. Make a list of the adults you can talk to so you can refer to when needed.

 Start thinking about situations which make you feel uncomfortable and begin to reflect how you can make a positive change.

The importance of exercise

Your body and mind are very important to you, they are the most valuable possessions you will ever have in your life.

People exercise every day for different reasons, for example:

Enjoyment, playing with friends, sports, at school, and sometimes also to help with negative feelings and illnesses.

Making daily exercise as part of your routine can have a very positive effect on your wellbeing.

It will boost your confidence, self-esteem, improve your energy levels, raise your fitness levels and give you better focus. These are just but a few examples of its benefits.

What exercise do you do and where?

The importance of exercise

How does exercising make you feel? Provide pictures as examples if you like.

The benefits of exercises include:

 Strengthening your heart

 Strengthening your bones and muscles

 When taking part in various team sports you can make new friends. Exercise can also help develop your confidence and make you feel really good about yourself.

 Exercise will increase your energy levels, which will help you concentrate throughout the day

 Exercise will also improve your fitness level

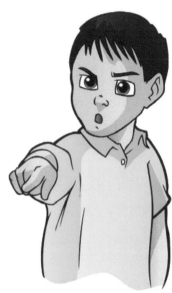

Over to you!

Can you name exercises or activities or different sports using every letter of the alphabet?

You can include any kind of: activity, sport or anything you see as a form of exercise.

A	Athletics
B	
C	
D	
E	
F	
G	
H	
I	

J	
K	
L	
M	
N	
O	
P	
Q	
R	
S	
T	
U	
V	
W	
X	
Y	
Z	

You only have one body, so make sure you look after it.

Lets workout!

Exercising with friends makes the experience so much more fun.

You can support each other, laugh together, and share the same experiences. Just remember that everyone has different abilities; just because they may not be as good as you at a specific exercise doesn't make them not good at all. If your friend is not as good as you in a certain activity, support them and help them to become better.

Here are some key words to use when exercising with your friends. "Well done! You are great! Keep going! You are doing very well! Fantastic! You are brilliant! I am so impressed with you and let's do this together!"

Use some positive words to help your friends complete their fitness circuits to the best of their ability.

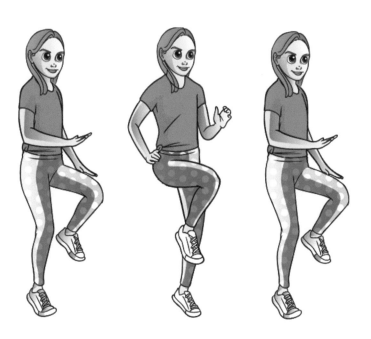

High Knees

Squats

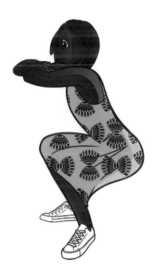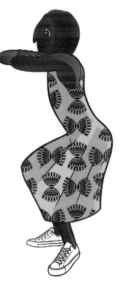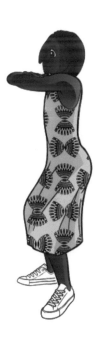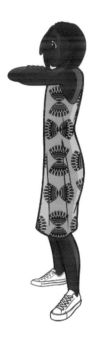

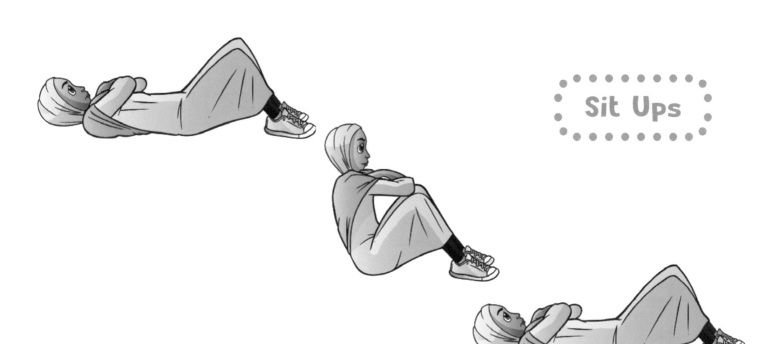

Sit Ups

Press Ups

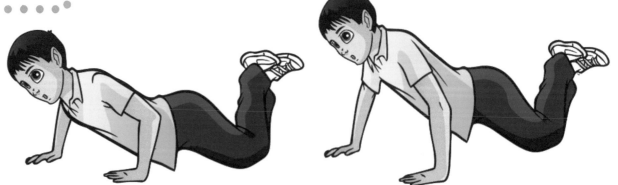

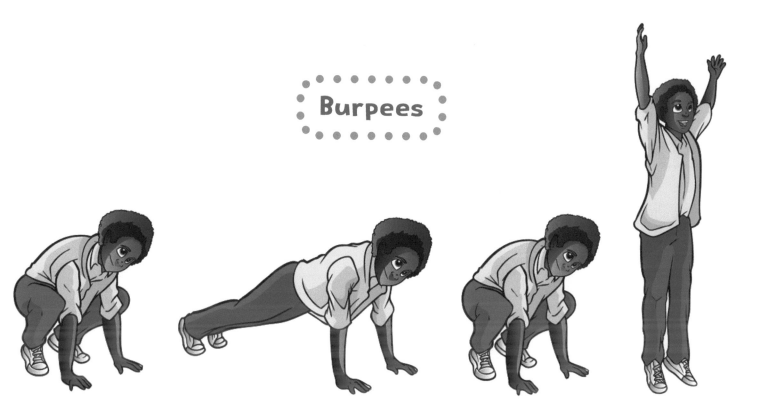

Burpees

It would be a great idea as part of your journey to become an Activ8 Hero, to pick one day of the week to complete this fitness test. Try and stick to this specific day as you can monitor your improvements more effectively. After every exercise, I want you to write in the box below how many times you done the exercise within the set time.

Fitness circuit: press ups, squats, burpees, sit ups, high knees - how many can you do in 45 seconds? Keep a log.

Exercise / Date	How many	How many?	How many	How many?	How many?	How many?	How many?	How many?
Press Ups								
Squats								
Burpeess								
Sit Ups								
High Knees								

If you have any restrictions which will stop you from taking part in this activity you can seek advice with an adult from a fitness professional to change the exercises.

Top Tips

 Practice the exercises throughout the week; this will help improve your score from the previous week.

 When you are doing the fitness test, ask someone to count how many times you do a particular exercise. We want you to give it your all and not have to think about this by yourself.

 Make sure you drink water in between the exercises.

 Take rest breaks in between the exercises.

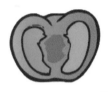

I love food! I enjoy every meal and I love food with a lot of flavours. We are surrounded by so many different kinds of food, from different nationalities, with different packaging and with so many different flavours.

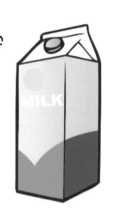

Some dishes have difficult names that are hard to remember, so here is a quick task: Can you name 5 different meals from different nationalities. Make sure you tell me where they are from.

Meal	Nationality

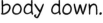

We should be eating natural foods every day to make sure we fuel our bodies correctly.

This will help us with our energy levels and allow us to complete tasks throughout the day to the best of our abilities.

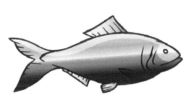

Think of a motor vehicle. It does not run if it doesn't have any petrol or if it has the wrong fuel. Look at food as a fuel for your body. If you haven't had anything to eat, you will not have energy for the day, and if you eat too many treats, it will slow your body down.

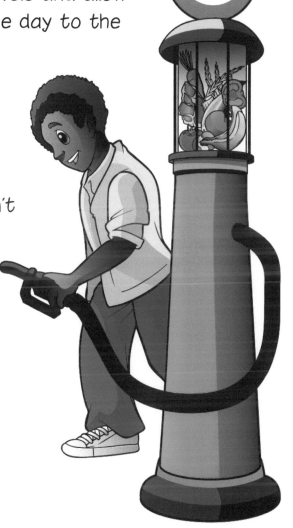

Food! Glorious Food!

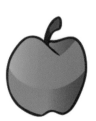

Can you make a list of all the natural foods that give you a lot of energy during the day and another list of foods that you can eat as a treat?

Fresh foods	Treat foods

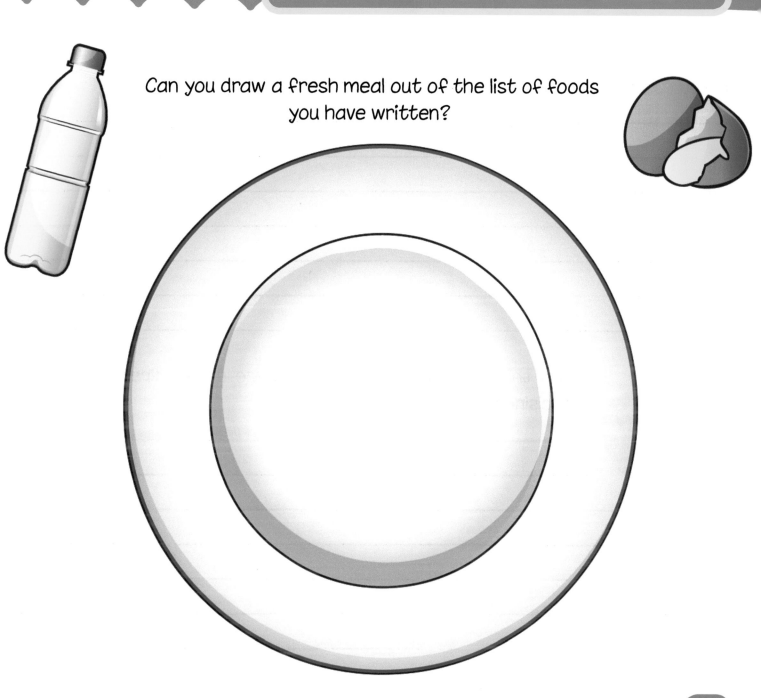

Can you draw a fresh meal out of the list of foods you have written?

Food! Glorious Food!

If you eat too many treats in a week, how does it make you feel?

_____

_____

_____

_____

_____

_____

How do think you would feel if you were eating fresh foods and exercising regularly?

_____

_____

_____

_____

_____

_____

The importance of sleep

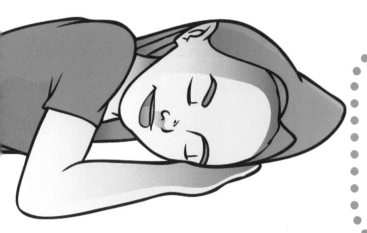

Sleep is very important. Sleep puts your body and mind to rest. We need sleep to keep us healthy, happy and to ensure we can have a positive and effective day by allowing us to do our best.

Sometimes, sleeping is not easy.

This is because we can easily be distracted by the objects around us.

It is very important to keep to regular sleeping patterns and to remove anything that can stop us from sleeping, so that we can wake up feeling our best.

I personally like to have everything written down on paper so that I can visualise my routines and remind myself what I need to do, even when I am supposed to go to bed!

The importance of sleep

What time should I go to sleep?	
What time do I need to wake up?	
What helps me to fall asleep?	
What prevents me from falling asleep?	

Did you know?

Sleep-walking tends to be a fairly normal part of your early sleep patterns.

Sleep helps with brain power.

Humans spent about a third of their lives sleeping.

Sleep increases your attention span.

People can take naps with their eyes open without even realising it.

A giraffe only needs 1.9 hours of sleep a day, whereas a brown bat needs 19.9 hours of sleep a day.

Well done, you did it!

Your first steps to Activ8ion is complete

It is such an achievement to have completed volume 1. You have officially taken you first step to Activ8tion.

You are now an Activ8 Hero. Remember, we can always improve and become better at what we do. We want you to keep practicing what you have learnt in this volume. Remember, practice makes progress.

We all look forward to seeing you in the next volume of **A step to Activ8tion** where we will take you on another fantastic journey.

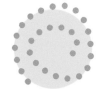
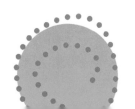

My daily reflective journal

Date:

What have I learned today?

What was the best part of my day?

What could I have done better today?

My goal for tomorrow is:

My daily reflective journal

Date:

What have I learned today?

What was the best part of my day?

What could I have done better today?

My goal for tomorrow is:

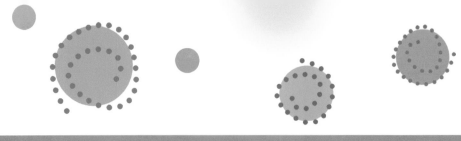

My daily reflective journal

Date:

What have I learned today?

What was the best part of my day?

What could I have done better today?

My goal for tomorrow is:

My daily reflective journal

Date:

What have I learned today?

What was the best part of my day?

What could I have done better today?

My goal for tomorrow is:

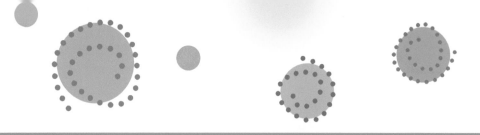

My daily reflective journal

Date:

What have I learned today?

What was the best part of my day?

What could I have done better today?

My goal for tomorrow is:

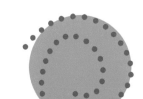

My daily reflective journal

Date:

What have I learned today?

What was the best part of my day?

What could I have done better today?

My goal for tomorrow is:

My daily reflective journal

Date:

What have I learned today?

What was the best part of my day?

What could I have done better today?

My goal for tomorrow is:

My daily reflective journal

Date:

What have I learned today?

What was the best part of my day?

What could I have done better today?

My goal for tomorrow is:

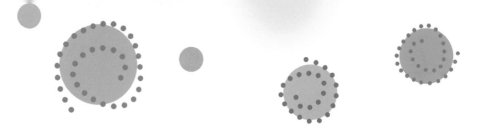

My daily reflective journal

Date:

What have I learned today?

What was the best part of my day?

What could I have done better today?

My goal for tomorrow is:

My daily reflective journal

Date:

What have I learned today?

What was the best part of my day?

What could I have done better today?

My goal for tomorrow is:

My daily reflective journal

Date:

What have I learned today?

What was the best part of my day?

What could I have done better today?

My goal for tomorrow is:

My daily reflective journal

Date:

What have I learned today?

What was the best part of my day?

What could I have done better today?

My goal for tomorrow is:

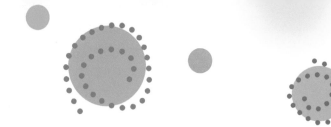

My daily reflective journal

Date:

What have I learned today?

What was the best part of my day?

What could I have done better today?

My goal for tomorrow is:

My daily reflective journal

Date:

What have I learned today?

What was the best part of my day?

What could I have done better today?

My goal for tomorrow is:

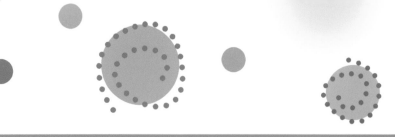

My daily reflective journal

Date:

What have I learned today?

What was the best part of my day?

What could I have done better today?

My goal for tomorrow is:

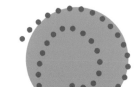

My daily reflective journal

Date:

What have I learned today?

What was the best part of my day?

What could I have done better today?

My goal for tomorrow is:

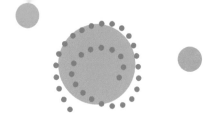

My daily reflective journal

Date:

What have I learned today?

What was the best part of my day?

What could I have done better today?

My goal for tomorrow is:

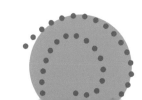

My daily reflective journal

Date:

What have I learned today?

What was the best part of my day?

What could I have done better today?

My goal for tomorrow is:

My daily reflective journal

Date:

What have I learned today?

What was the best part of my day?

What could I have done better today?

My goal for tomorrow is:

My daily reflective journal

Date:

What have I learned today?

What was the best part of my day?

What could I have done better today?

My goal for tomorrow is:

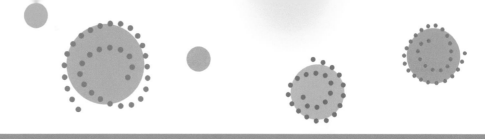

My daily reflective journal

Date:

What have I learned today?

What was the best part of my day?

What could I have done better today?

My goal for tomorrow is:

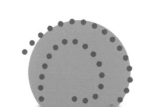

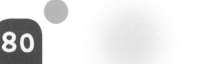

My daily reflective journal

Date:

What have I learned today?

What was the best part of my day?

What could I have done better today?

My goal for tomorrow is:

My daily reflective journal

Date:

What have I learned today?

What was the best part of my day?

What could I have done better today?

My goal for tomorrow is:

My daily reflective journal

Date:

What have I learned today?

What was the best part of my day?

What could I have done better today?

My goal for tomorrow is:

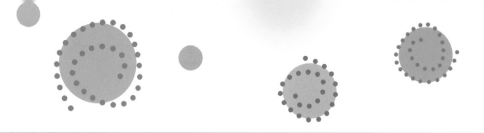

My daily reflective journal

Date:

What have I learned today?

What was the best part of my day?

What could I have done better today?

My goal for tomorrow is:

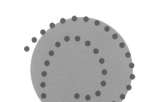

My daily reflective journal

Date:

What have I learned today?

What was the best part of my day?

What could I have done better today?

My goal for tomorrow is:

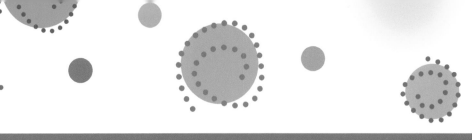

My daily reflective journal

Date:

What have I learned today?

What was the best part of my day?

What could I have done better today?

My goal for tomorrow is:

My daily reflective journal

Date:

What have I learned today?

What was the best part of my day?

What could I have done better today?

My goal for tomorrow is:

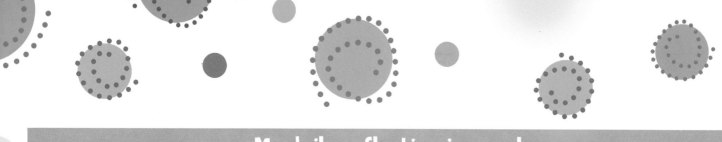

My daily reflective journal

Date:

What have I learned today?

What was the best part of my day?

What could I have done better today?

My goal for tomorrow is:

My daily reflective journal

Date:

What have I learned today?

What was the best part of my day?

What could I have done better today?

My goal for tomorrow is:

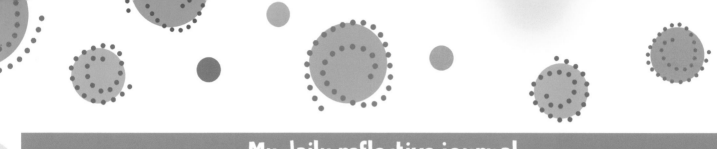

My daily reflective journal

Date:

What have I learned today?

What was the best part of my day?

What could I have done better today?

My goal for tomorrow is:

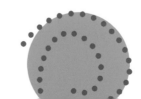

My daily reflective journal

Date:

What have I learned today?

What was the best part of my day?

What could I have done better today?

My goal for tomorrow is:

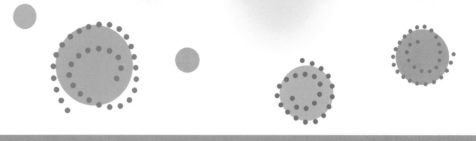

My daily reflective journal

Date:

What have I learned today?

What was the best part of my day?

What could I have done better today?

My goal for tomorrow is:

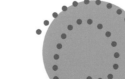

My daily reflective journal

Date:

What have I learned today?

What was the best part of my day?

What could I have done better today?

My goal for tomorrow is:

My daily reflective journal

Date:

What have I learned today?

What was the best part of my day?

What could I have done better today?

My goal for tomorrow is:

My daily reflective journal

Date:

What have I learned today?

What was the best part of my day?

What could I have done better today?

My goal for tomorrow is:

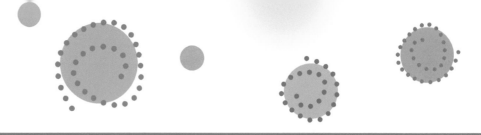

My daily reflective journal

Date:

What have I learned today?

What was the best part of my day?

What could I have done better today?

My goal for tomorrow is:

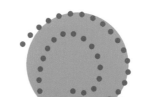

My daily reflective journal

Date:

What have I learned today?

What was the best part of my day?

What could I have done better today?

My goal for tomorrow is:

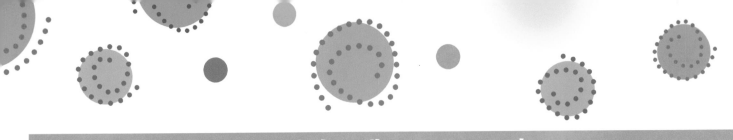

My daily reflective journal

Date:

What have I learned today?

What was the best part of my day?

What could I have done better today?

My goal for tomorrow is:

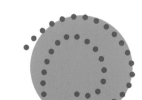

My daily reflective journal

Date:

What have I learned today?

What was the best part of my day?

What could I have done better today?

My goal for tomorrow is:

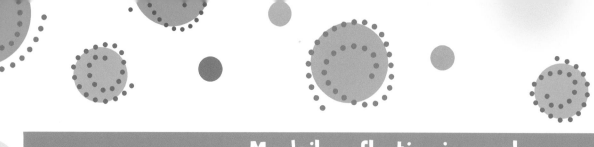

My daily reflective journal

Date:

What have I learned today?

What was the best part of my day?

What could I have done better today?

My goal for tomorrow is:

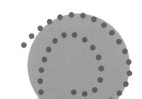

My daily reflective journal

Date:

What have I learned today?

What was the best part of my day?

What could I have done better today?

My goal for tomorrow is:

My daily reflective journal

Date:

What have I learned today?

What was the best part of my day?

What could I have done better today?

My goal for tomorrow is:

My daily reflective journal

Date:

What have I learned today?

What was the best part of my day?

What could I have done better today?

My goal for tomorrow is:

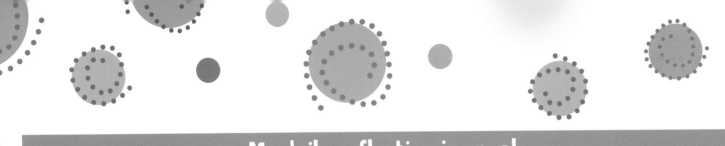

My daily reflective journal

Date:

What have I learned today?

What was the best part of my day?

What could I have done better today?

My goal for tomorrow is:

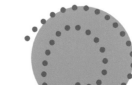

My daily reflective journal

Date:

What have I learned today?

What was the best part of my day?

What could I have done better today?

My goal for tomorrow is:

My daily reflective journal

Date:

What have I learned today?

What was the best part of my day?

What could I have done better today?

My goal for tomorrow is:

My daily reflective journal

Date:

What have I learned today?

What was the best part of my day?

What could I have done better today?

My goal for tomorrow is:

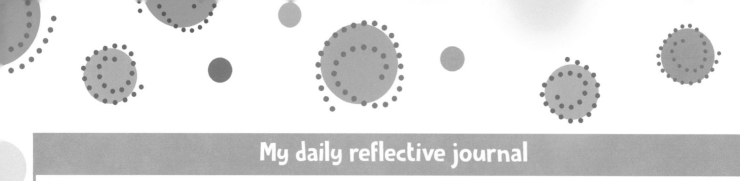

My daily reflective journal

Date:

What have I learned today?

What was the best part of my day?

What could I have done better today?

My goal for tomorrow is:

My daily reflective journal

Date:

What have I learned today?

What was the best part of my day?

What could I have done better today?

My goal for tomorrow is:

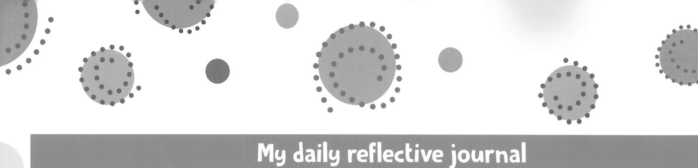

My daily reflective journal

Date:

What have I learned today?

What was the best part of my day?

What could I have done better today?

My goal for tomorrow is:

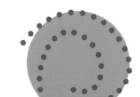

My daily reflective journal

Date:

What have I learned today?

What was the best part of my day?

What could I have done better today?

My goal for tomorrow is:

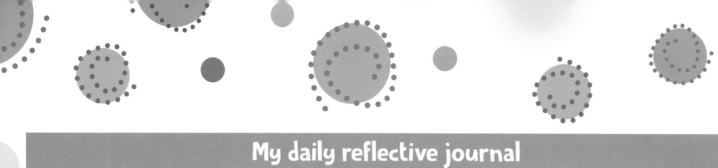

My daily reflective journal

Date:

What have I learned today?

What was the best part of my day?

What could I have done better today?

My goal for tomorrow is:

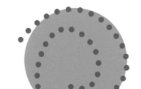

My daily reflective journal

Date:

What have I learned today?

What was the best part of my day?

What could I have done better today?

My goal for tomorrow is:

My daily reflective journal

Date:

What have I learned today?

What was the best part of my day?

What could I have done better today?

My goal for tomorrow is:

My daily reflective journal

Date:

What have I learned today?

What was the best part of my day?

What could I have done better today?

My goal for tomorrow is:

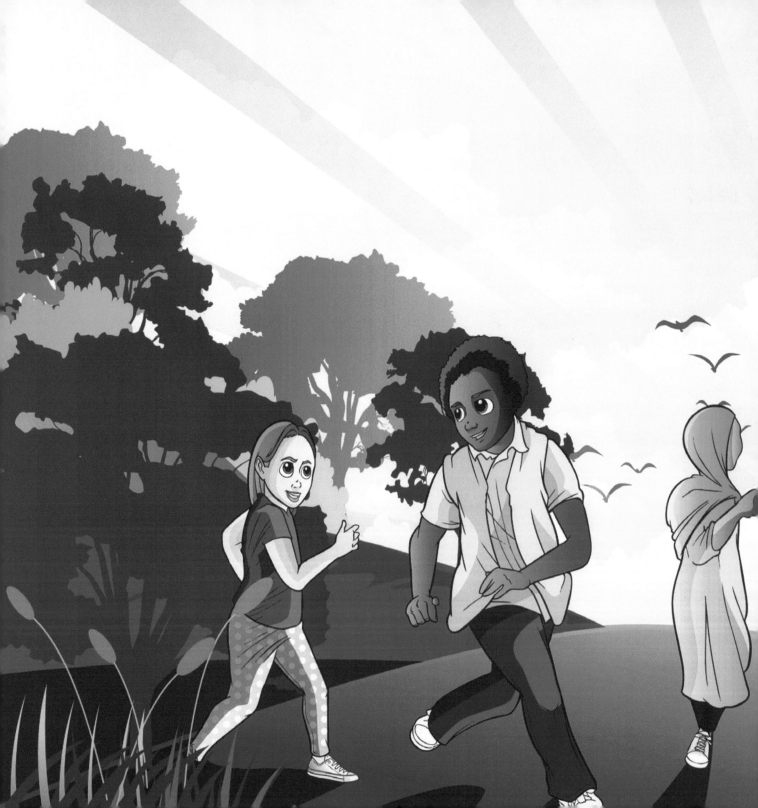

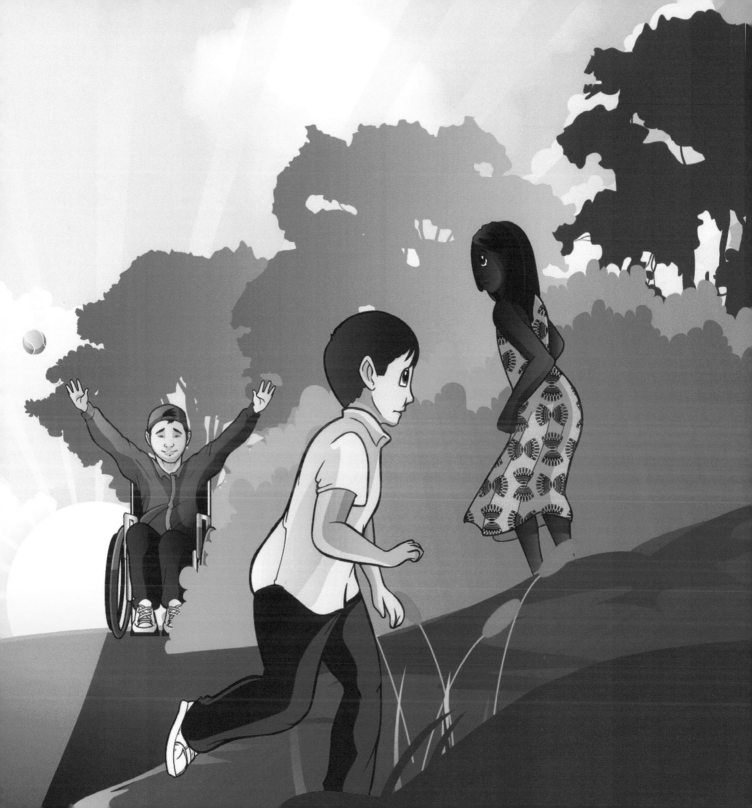